DIABETES DIET
Blood Sugar Control with Diet and Herbal Medicines

Grace C. Benson

Copyright

Table of Content

CHAPTER ONE

Introduction

Diabetes is a global medical condition, affecting millions of people of all ages worldwide. It is a disease that results from the inability of the pancreas to produce enough insulin for body use or when the body lacks the capacity to use the insulin produced. Insulin is the hormone produced to monitor the blood glucose level. Where the blood sugar is left uncontrolled could result to adverse damage to many body organs/systems. This condition is called hyperglycaemia.

The yearly increase in mortality rate worldwide has become a concern to reckon with. In 2014, research recorded 8.4% diabetic patients between 18-40 years old. In 2019, the number increased to 48% record, causing 1.5 million deaths of patients before the age of 70 years. Another record estimated 20% cardiovascular deaths caused by diabetes.

Symptoms of diabetes could either be quickly noticeable or hidden for years before been noticed. Such hidden cases are much dangerous than the former. The quickly noticeable cases indicates Type 1 Diabetes, while the latter indicates Type 2 Diabetes. To prevent the worst scenario of Type 2 Diabetes can be prevented by undertaking early diagnosis, which involve regular checkups and blood tests by your doctor.

Lifestyle modifications are the approaches to preventing the disaster of diabetes. These lifestyle habits include: eating diet devoid of sugar and saturated fats, regular exercise, avoid smoking cigarette, etc.

The treatment approach for diabetes is based on the result of the diagnosis. Each type of diabetes diagnosed has its own version of medication/treatment.

Signs and Symptoms

The signs and symptoms of diabetes differs in occurrence base on the type. Type 1 diabetes, the symptoms are quickly noticeable while type 2 diabetes, the symptoms can be hidden for years before being noticed. This type should be treated full caution.

Symptoms of this medical condition – diabetes include:

- Frequent urination
- Blurred vision
- Feeling too thirsty often
- Fatigue
- Unwanted loss of weight

As the symptoms progresses or left untreated for a period of time, they begin to damage blood vessels in the heart, eyes, kidneys and nerves. This is why people with diabetes are readily susceptible to other diseases attack such as heart attack, stroke, and vision loss and kidney failure.

The Mechanism of Insulin Production and Secretion

Insulin is an amino acid and is highly conserved in all mammals. One insulin in one mammal is almost the same biologically active in another mammal. This is why today, patients are sometimes treated with insulin extracted from pigs' pancreas.

Biosynthesis

In the beta cells, insulin is synthesized in greater quantities in the pancreas, where the insulin – mRNA is configured in a single chain called preproinsulin. The removal of its peptide (an inherent signal) during mixture into the endoplasmic reticulum creates proinsulin.

The proinsulin is a compact substance composed of three domains:

1. An amino-terminal B chain
2. A carboxy-terminal A chain and
3. An attaching/linking peptide in the middle – the C peptide

The proinsuline is exposed to many specific endopeptidases within the walls of endoplasmic reticulum. This leads to the formation of mature form of insulin. This is the last of synthesis as insulin and free C peptides are arranged in the Golgi bodies and sent to the secretory granules accumulated in the cytoplasm.

Insulin Secretion

Insulin is secreted from the beta cells upon adequate stimulation by a process – exocytosis. The insulin is then made to diffuse into the blood vessels of the pancreas alongside the C peptides.

This is the process flow for insulin synthesis and secretion.

CHAPTER TWO

Types of Diabetes

The knowledge of the different types of diabetes that could impair your blood usage and regulation of sugar is startup guide to preventing their occurrences. There three types of diabetes, namely:

1. Type 1 diabetes
2. Type 2 diabetes and
3. Gestational diabetes

Now, we shall consider the potential causes of the three diabetes, their individual symptoms and treatment approaches.

Type 1 Diabetes

Type 1 diabetes results when the immune system attacks and impairs the beta cells that produces insulin in the pancreas. The potential attacker makes an autoimmune disease.

Till date, the cause of this beta cell uproar is yet unknown, but has a link with genetic ad environmental factors.

Signs and symptoms

- Weight loss – diabetic ketoacidosis
- Retarded healing of wounds

Treatment

Since the beta cells is damaged, insulin is injected into the patient's skin. The insulin are in different types available in variations of onset, peak and duration.

Insulin pump can also be used as external device worn outside the body to release calculated amount of insulin.

Constant daily monitoring of your blood sugar level is necessary to keep you from danger. Medications are also available to manage other underlying conditions such as cholesterol, high blood pressure, etc.

Type 2 Diabetes

This type of diabetes is like a hidden snake waiting to chop off a passing grasshopper. Type 2 diabetes begins by resisting the free secretion of insulin, making it difficult for the body to use insulin efficiently. The pancreas is continuously stimulated to secrete more insulin until it loses all its capacity to secrete more, which then results to high blood sugar.

Signs Symptoms

- Discolored patches in skin of the armpit and neck
- Pain or numbness in your feet

Causes

There are no actual causes yet, but are linked to sedentary lifestyle, obesity

Treatment

Type 2 diabetes can be treated or even reversed with consistent and well-pragrammed exercise and healthy diet. It can as well be tackled with some medications, namely: metformin (Glumetza, Glucophage, Fortamet, Riomet). The mechanism of these drugs is geared towards reducing glucose production in the liver.

Gestational Diabetes

Gestational diabetes is the result of insulin-blocking hormone prevalent during pregnancy. Because it only occur during pregnancy, some refer to it as pregnancy diabetes.

Just like the other types of diabetes, gestational diabetes affects your body's glucose integrity by raising the level of your blood sugar, which consequently affects your pregnancy and health of your baby. One way of avoiding this is, eating healthy diet. Foods that are more of fruits or Mediterranean, exercise and medication where necessary. By trying to control your blood sugar level, you protect the health of your child.

Symptoms

This type of diabetes often has its symptoms unnoticeable, but some signs include:

- Increased thirst
- Frequent urination

Causes

Numerous research have been carried out as to what exactly causes gestational diabetes, but nothing exactly has been discovered. However, excess weight was found to be a contributing factor.

Several hormones are produced in the body to process and keep blood sugar level in check, but this is usually inhibited during pregnancy, making it difficult for the body process its sugar level. This leads to increase in blood sugar level.

Complications

Increased sugar level can interfere with your health and that of your child if not properly managed or controlled. Some risk complications for your baby during this period include:

- Excessive birth weight: if blood sugar goes uncontrolled, it causes the birth of too large babies that weighs 9 pounds or more.
- Early (preterm) birth: uncontrolled sugar level can lead to early child

delivery or the recommendation of it.

- Severe breathing difficulties: premature babies – babies born before their time often experience difficulty breathing (respiratory distress syndrome).
- Low blood sugar (hyperglycemia): often low blood sugar results in babies born prematurely. This causes seizures in the baby.

Prevention

Just as the actual cause of gestational diabetes is yet unknown, so are the preventive measures. But suggested recommendations have been found to be helpful. Some of which include:

- Practicing eating healthy diets. Your choice of diet should be fruits, vegetables. Foods high in fiber content and low in fats and calories.

- Keep fit. Regular engagement in simple workouts before and during pregnant can help prevent gestational diabetes. 30minutes road walk, bike riding, lap swimming, etc are some simple workouts you can keep to.

- Keep healthy weight before pregnant. Managing your weight through simple exercises and healthy diet, such as fruits and vegetables before getting pregnant, can help prevent gestational diabetes caused by excess weight.

- Avoid gaining more weight than necessary before and during pregnancy period.

Treatment

Conscious management of your blood sugar level will help keep you and your child healthy. Recommendable treatments for gestational diabetes include:

- Lifestyle modification: this include eating healthy diet which must not exceed or exclude fruits, vegetables, whole grains, and lean protein. Also, staying active by engaging in some regular physical activities play important roles in helping avoid gestational diabetes during pregnancy
- Blood sugar monitory: your doctor will recommend you check your blood sugar level frequently, say, 4 times a day to make sure your level does not exceed the normal.

- Medication: where the two above options does not give good result, you may be injected with insulin to lower your blood sugar. Most pregnant women need this option to maintain the required blood sugar level.

CHAPTER THREE

Diabetes Diet

Diabetes as a global health epidemic is a chronic metabolic disorder characterized by elevated blood sugar levels, resulting from the body's inability to produce or effectively use insulin. This condition affects millions of individuals worldwide, posing significant health challenges and economic burdens. Diabetes comes in two primary forms: Type 1 and Type 2.

Type 1 diabetes typically manifests in childhood or adolescence and is an autoimmune condition where the body's immune system mistakenly destroys insulin-producing beta cells in the pancreas. This form requires lifelong insulin therapy.

On the other hand, Type 2 diabetes, often linked to obesity and lifestyle factors, is the most prevalent form and can develop at any age. It results from insulin resistance or decreased insulin production. Lifestyle modifications, including a balanced diet and regular exercise, play a crucial role in its management.

Left uncontrolled, diabetes can lead to severe complications, such as cardiovascular disease, kidney problems, neuropathy, and blindness. Early detection, proper management, and increased awareness are essential in the fight against this silent epidemic.

A diabetes diet plays an important role in managing blood sugar levels and overall health for individuals with diabetes. I know you would like know some of these healthy regimen. Here's a list of key dietary components and their detailed explanations:

1. **Carbohydrates:**
   - *Complex Carbohydrates:* These include whole grains (brown rice, quinoa, whole wheat bread), legumes (beans, lentils), and starchy vegetables (sweet potatoes). They release glucose into the bloodstream slowly, preventing rapid spikes in blood sugar.
   - *Fiber:* High-fiber foods like vegetables, fruits, whole grains, and nuts help stabilize blood sugar levels by slowing down the absorption of glucose. Fiber also supports digestive health and can aid in weight management.

- *Sugars and Simple Carbohydrates:* Limit added sugars and refined carbohydrates like sugary drinks, candies, and white bread. These can cause rapid blood sugar spikes and should be consumed sparingly.

2. **Proteins:**

- Lean protein sources like skinless poultry, fish, tofu, legumes, and low-fat dairy can help regulate blood sugar and provide essential nutrients. Protein also promotes satiety and can aid in weight control.

3. **Fats:**

- *Healthy Fats:* Include sources of unsaturated fats like avocados, olive oil, nuts, and fatty fish (salmon, mackerel).

These fats can improve insulin sensitivity and support cardiovascular health.

- *Limit Saturated and Trans Fats:* Reduce saturated fats from red meat and full-fat dairy, as well as trans fats from processed and fried foods. High intake of these fats can increase the risk of heart disease.

4. **Portion Control:**

- Controlling portion sizes is crucial to managing calorie intake and blood sugar levels. Measuring food, using smaller plates, and practicing mindful eating can help with portion control.

5. **Meal Timing:**

- Consistent meal timing helps maintain stable blood sugar levels. Eating at regular intervals throughout the day, including healthy snacks if necessary, can prevent extreme fluctuations.

6. **Monitoring Carbohydrate Intake:**
   - Carbohydrate counting allows individuals to track and manage their carb intake accurately, helping with insulin dosing and blood sugar control.

7. **Glycemic Index (GI):**
   - Foods with a low GI release glucose slowly and can help stabilize blood sugar levels. These include most non-starchy vegetables, legumes, and whole grains.

8. **Hydration:**
   - Staying well-hydrated is essential for overall health. Water is the best choice, and sugary drinks should be avoided.

9. **Alcohol:**
   - If consumed, alcohol should be limited and consumed with caution as it can affect blood sugar levels and interact with diabetes medications.

10. **Individualized Plans:**
   - It's important to remember that there is no one-size-fits-all diabetes diet. Individual dietary plans should be developed in consultation with a healthcare provider or registered dietitian based on a

person's specific needs, preferences, and goals.

The importance, the need to inculcate healthy ad balanced diet into your meal routines cannot be overstated. A well-balanced diabetes diet focuses on whole, unprocessed foods, emphasizes portion control, and is tailored to an individual's unique needs. It should also be part of a broader diabetes management plan that includes regular physical activity and ongoing monitoring of blood sugar levels.

Herbal Medicines for Diabetes

Herbs have been used for centuries in various traditional medicine systems to complement diabetes management. These herbal medications has been proven by research to work as well as the conventional treatment while into consideration the varied responses in different individuals. While they should not replace conventional medical treatments, some herbs may offer potential benefits for individuals with diabetes. Here are some herbs often explored in this context, along with detailed explanations:

1. **Cinnamon (Cinnamomum verum or Cinnamomum cassia):** Cinnamon contains bioactive compounds that can improve insulin sensitivity and help lower blood sugar levels. Some studies suggest that daily consumption of cinnamon may reduce fasting blood sugar levels in individuals with type 2 diabetes. You can add cinnamon to your diet by sprinkling it on

oatmeal, yogurt, or including it in herbal teas.

2. **Fenugreek (Trigonella foenum-graecum):** Fenugreek seeds are rich in soluble fiber and compounds that may slow down the absorption of sugar in the digestive tract. Research indicates that fenugreek supplements or seeds may help lower blood sugar levels and improve insulin sensitivity. You can incorporate fenugreek seeds into your diet by soaking and consuming them or adding them to curries and stews.

3. **Bitter Melon (Momordica charantia):** Bitter melon, a tropical vegetable, has been used traditionally to manage diabetes. It contains substances that may mimic the action of insulin and help regulate blood sugar. Bitter melon

can be consumed as a vegetable or taken in supplement form.

4. **Gymnema Sylvestre:** Gymnema is an herb native to India and has been used in Ayurvedic medicine to support diabetes management. It may reduce sugar absorption in the intestines and enhance insulin function. Gymnema is available in supplement form and may help control sugar cravings.

5. **Ginger (Zingiber officinale):** Ginger has anti-inflammatory properties and may improve insulin sensitivity. Studies suggest that ginger supplementation can lead to modest reductions in blood sugar levels. You can incorporate ginger into your diet by adding it to dishes or brewing ginger tea.

6. **Aloe Vera:** Aloe vera gel, extracted from the inner leaf, may help lower blood sugar levels in people with type 2 diabetes. It is available in juice or supplement form.

Before incorporating herbs into your diabetes management plan, it's crucial to consult with a healthcare professional or registered herbalist. They can provide guidance on appropriate dosages, potential interactions with medications, and monitor your progress. It's essential to remember that while herbs may offer some benefits, they should not replace prescribed diabetes treatments but rather complement them as part of a comprehensive healthcare strategy. Regular monitoring of blood sugar levels and lifestyle modifications remain fundamental in diabetes management.

Conclusion

The journey through the pages of this book has been both enlightening and empowering. We've uncovered the intricate scenarios of diabetes, discovering its various types, each with its unique challenges and implications for those living with the condition.

The primary roles of diet in managing diabetes cannot be overstated. Through meticulous examination, we've seen how the right dietary choices can be a potent tool in blood sugar control, and hence, a hope and improved quality of life to countless individuals. From the importance of managing carbohydrate intake to incorporating fiber-rich foods, we've uncovered topnotch dietary strategies that can make a world of difference.

Moreover, the exploration of herbs as complementary therapies for diabetes provided a glimpse into the fascinating world of natural remedies. Herbs like bitter melon, fenugreek, and cinnamon have been used for centuries to help regulate blood sugar levels.

A newfound understanding of diabetes, its nuances, and the empowering knowledge of how diet and herbs can be harnessed to manage this condition effectively welcome fulfilled and promising lives.

It is my hope that the insights gained here will serve as an inspiration for those facing the daily challenges of diabetes, offering them the tools they need to live healthier and more fulfilling lives.